CW01551743

# The Voices That Haunt Us

To better days.

## About the author

Dave is a Northern Irish man in exile in England. He lives in York with his wife and two young sons, who are the best thing in his life.

After working for 15 years in church work with a short foray into working in healthcare, Dave has taken a slight career pivot to work in the charity sector.

He is passionate about seeing people discover themselves and to reach their potential and enjoys being alongside people of all ages and helping them do just that.

Dave tries to write short books as he finds that he rarely finishes a book which goes beyond 120 pages despite often being unable to put them down before that point.

Dave loves being in nature with his boys, drinking good or bad coffee with friends, a good rioja and baking bread.

If you want to chat to him, he's on twitter @davemagill and, against his better judgement, has am author page on Facebook.

You can also get in touch through his website, www.davemagill.com

# 1. David Robert Magill

That's me. David Robert Magill. It's been on bank cards and business cards, office doors and marriage certificates; David Robert Magill. Me. Those letters on their own are meaningless but, if the world was a solid-state drive or a Bruce Almighty sized filing cabinet, my life would be filed under David Robert Magill.

My name is the label that connects everything that I've ever encountered or thought or said or done. Every one of my achievements rests underneath those 17 letters, marked into the report card of my life. I am the common denominator in every moment of joy and every moment of pain. The fragments of my existence are bound up in my name, they are the story of who I am, held together by my life.

When people hear my name some will be filled with, pride (Hello, Mum, and Dad). Others will hear my name and remember the times I let them down, they'll be angry at a slight or pain for which I am responsible. Others will think of me as an ex, or an almost-boyfriend, some of them with a 'what if' and others with a 'thank God.' My name heard by every person I know will bring a mix of opinions and memories based on very few or very many moments we shared together. I am all these things at once, based upon the person I was in the moments I spent with people.

My name, our names, are loaded with meaning, much more than any word in any language. Our names tell stories to those who hear them spoken, and most importantly they tell stories to ourselves. It's those stories that I'm writing about in this book. The narratives, which we weave together from the events of our lives, are how we define ourselves. We are responsible for every scene, every plotline and we control all of the dialogue. Every voice in these stories is our own voice, at times repeating what we have heard, sometimes with exact precision, other times with embellished or blemished details that change their meaning in our lives.

What are the stories that we tell ourselves about who we are? Which voices are speaking the story of our name, of our identity, and why are we listening to them? Are they good for us or are they slowly tearing us apart?

For the last few years, and most probably much longer than that, I've been fighting with my own mind. I was diagnosed with severe stress and anxiety in September 2016 and have since been on various treatments, both therapy, and medication. I am sure that my diagnosis could have been the same at least a decade earlier. In retrospect, the symptoms were all there but in my mid to late twenties, I still had enough distraction or vigour or luck to keep going. I was able to mask the battle that was happening in my head and continue to make my way through life. At 36, however, the wheels came off, and my ability to suffer any longer reached zero. My body could no longer sustain itself as the storm within my brain raged. My health began to collapse as my body began to manifest the effects of anxiety, stress, depression, and the exhaustion of battling all three.

I had been fighting for a worthy cause, my own self-worth, but I was fighting alone and with the wrong weaponry. I was never going to win on my own with the tools available to me, at best I might hold my ground from time to time. So, exhausted I surrendered to my own demands and admitted the truth. I was ill, I was mentally ill, and I needed help. I needed it to come quickly.

It's been hard to admit that to myself. It's been hard to admit that I'm mentally ill, haunted by my own thoughts, and kept level by medication. I'd painted a picture of myself in my head as someone for whom that kind of thing could never be possible. I was a strong and brave man, rarely intimidated by any situation, and able to keep a cool head under pressure. I had created the persona of a laid back, happy go lucky guy who could deal with anything thrown at him with great poise and wisdom.

It was hard to admit that I regularly (and less regularly now) could feel my body slip into the symptoms of panic as my mind fell silent, refusing to bring calm or solution to the moment. As my body tensed up, my chest tightened, my breath turning shallower as my heart raced, my mind felt like it was on mute. I was panicking but I was silent, it was like an out of body experience. At times I felt like I was dying at the same time as being completely still.

It was hard to admit that I was throwing up before the most innocuous of occasions and that often my chest felt so tight that I was sure that my lungs were being crushed between my ribs. Every day for a year, I wretched on my knees in the bathroom before walking to work. Anxiety had found a home in my mind and it was getting worse. It was hard to admit it but it was the truth.

I was hiding all of this from everyone as best I could. The effort of suffering in secret made things worse. On top of being anxious about work, failing as a father, money, how I was viewed, my health, and the unexplained sense of dread that was a constant background noise to my day, I was now anxious about how I could hide my symptoms. I was managing mental illness at the same time as managing a cover-up. It was exhausting.

Anxiety will probably be a part of my life for the long term. I have made choices to do things that minimise its impact, but there are days, like today, 8th July 2020, that I feel like my body is fizzing, my mind can't find a second of stillness and I need to scream. I find myself caught in a loop of imagining and dismantling imminent catastrophes. On days like this one, the unexplained sense of dread is no longer a low background hum, it thuds in my head like a bass drum. There are days, like today, that I'm afraid for no reason that I can name, but worry has rested heavily on my shoulders since I woke up at 7:25 am. I am tense and I am tetchy. I wish I could rest.

When I was told by my GP that I was mentally ill, I decided to live my illness in public. My first reaction to being told that I was ill was shame, then denial, then retreat. I slept for a long time. I slept the majority of every day for three weeks. I'd exhausted myself, fighting with my own brain rather than fighting for it. I was empty. After those three weeks, I decided to be public about what I suffer, and suffer is not too strong a word. If I was initially ashamed it was because a societal stigma about mental illness had found this way into my beliefs. I had absorbed the idea that those who need help with their minds are weak snowflakes, unable to cope with the real world. The truth, of course, is that being able to function at all in this world whilst being plagued by one's own mind is incredibly strong and brave. I thought that perhaps my story could stop someone else feeling the shame that I did. The feeling of not being alone in our pain, or that someone else knows how it feels, can give us a much-needed boost to keep fighting.

That's why I am writing this little book. I don't know if there will be solutions for things, but I will share the things I've found helpful, but what I do know is that if you've suffered some of the things that I suffer that you will feel seen. You will feel less alone because you'll know someone else hasn't just been there, but are probably there right now. I know this will happen because that's been my experience with those who live their pain in public, the reading helps me.

Remember I am not the first, nor last to walk this trail, and I don't walk it alone.

There are many voices that echo in my mind, and I assume the minds of other people, that are destructive to our mental health. Voices of shame, expectation, and disappointment that haunt us in our most quiet moments. There are memories of loss or feelings of inadequacy that rob us of moments of joy as we move through the world. Sometimes these voices shout loudly over any other voices and sometimes they are still and quiet but no less destructive.

I realised about a year ago that every voice in my head that tells me I'm less or that I should be afraid is actually my own voice. Every negative word that my mind speaks over my identity is spoken by me. Sure, I may be borrowing the words of others who have criticised or abused me, but the continual speaking of those words over my life is from my own consciousness. I am the one speaking in the voices that haunt me the most.

It follows that if I, albeit subconsciously, am bringing these thoughts to my mind that I can also silence them or react to them with other thoughts that speak positivity and hope. I am not responsible for what enters my mind but I can take responsibility for how I respond to those thoughts. I can work to train my mind to respond with hopeful truth to every negative thought I have about myself.

Haunted is a strong word. I realise that it feels like an exaggeration but late at night when my mind is filled with shame or fear, or when I fail to make a decision because I am anxious about the outcomes, I feel haunted by my own mind. The hardest part of this haunting is that I know that the circular thoughts and rabbit warrens are bad for my health, yet they feel true and somehow alluring at the time. Negative and self-critical thinking has a strangely addictive quality. The words they speak draw me towards the rocks like Siren song, serenading Jason, and his Argonauts in an attempt to lead him to destruction. I must then, paint myself as Orpheus and find a louder, more beautiful song that keeps me moving forward; a song that speaks uplifting truth to my mind and saves me from the rocks.

I hope you find this little book helpful in some way. I've tried to keep this book short for two reasons. When my anxiety is bad I find reading difficult and exhausting. I also hate books that are long for no reason. I hope it's an easy read.

I hope it isn't too heavy and that there are laughs amongst the solemnity. I hope, that in reading of my battle with my own mind, you feel less alone in your own battles. I hope you feel solidarity and comfort in knowing that change is possible. I hope you find a louder and more beautiful song. I hope that one day we can all find peace.

## 2. Loneliness

Loneliness is a killer. It quietly sneaks into our lives and pushes us to the edge of what we can handle. The organsiation, Campaign Against Loneliness recently shared a list of some hard-hitting statistics on loneliness, here are a handful of examples[1]:

-   It is estimated that by 2025/26 that 2 million over 50s in the UK will be experiencing chronic loneliness, an increase of 49% on the previous decade (Age UK 2018, All The Lonely People).
-   Research by The British Red Cross and Coop reveal that 9 million UK adults of all ages always, or almost always experience feelings of loneliness.

---

[1]
https://www.campaigntoendloneliness.org/the-facts-on-loneliness/

- Action for Children have released evidence that 43% of all young adults (17-25) have experienced loneliness and under half of those surveyed say they feel loved.
- 50% of disabled people say that they often feel lonely.

When the UK national press report on loneliness they use words like 'epidemic' or 'health crisis' and I have often considered these to be deliberate hyperbole chosen in order to sell papers. However, having read some studies by charities and universities it may be that loneliness is even more of a problem for our society than this language suggests. Loneliness is a health concern, it is literally killing people, through physical and mental health issues. Loneliness drives people to their deaths by suicide. It exacerbates other health issues and, in keeping people removed from community, stops thousands of people from getting help and support that they deserve and need.

Loneliness is measurable and real, but in this chapter, I want to draw a slight distinction between the voice of loneliness and the loneliness that these statistics are speaking of. For the sake of that distinction, I'd like to label the loneliness of these statistics and studies and isolation, i.e. the physical state of being alone. Isolation is a consistent and unchosen lack of human contact. Isolation is at epidemic proportions but so also is the voice of loneliness, that is, the voice in our head that tells us we are alone.

The phrase is a cliché, well worn of its original efficacy, but the feeling of being alone in a crowded room is a deeply painful experience. It is also an experience with which I am all too familiar. A few years ago my wife and I were part of a church which held smaller group meetings on a weeknight. These were held in a church member's home and were very relaxed and welcoming affairs with coffee, cake and conversation (Christians love alliteration). We would go faithfully every week, we would receive regular WhatsApp messages from the group. There were in-jokes and shared memories. We would belly laugh recalling the time that someone had embarrassed themselves and other times we would listen in support as someone would share of their job loss or bereavement. These were the very definition of good people, generously giving themselves to others.

From the outside, my membership of that small group must have looked life-giving but the reality was that every week on the drive home we would have the same conversation in the car. I would leave the group feeling that I did not belong, that I was not welcome. I was convinced that I was not liked, nevermind loved. I was sure that people found me annoying or ill-informed. The best I could accept was that I was tolerated by them. My mind had turned on me, I could not see the good in my life through fear and the pain which followed it.

I was in a group of people who cared deeply for one another and yet I felt alone. I was consistently in a room of 15 people whom I knew by name. I knew their jobs and the names of their children. I knew their preference for tea or coffee and the details of their most recent exercise regimes but I felt lonely when I was with them. This often made little sense to my long-suffering wife. She could see that those people cared about me, to her eyes it was unmissable, but I couldn't believe it. She always had a list of evidence that they cared, all of which was factual, but it made little difference, I was lonely in a crowded room.

I must say again at this point that the people in that room were and are wonderful people who did care deeply about me and who showed that care in many ways. They showed up for us many times when we needed support. They called and texted to check-in. They are kind and loving people. My experience of loneliness had little to do with them or their actions. It wouldn't have mattered what they did, I was incapable of feeling it. My experience of loneliness was about the voice of loneliness in my head and not about them at all. I was haunted by a voice that told me I didn't belong, a voice that told me I didn't fit in. That voice had changed how I acted and the behaviours that followed caused me to magnify my own feelings of seclusion.

One of the thoughts that would come up in our conversations on that weekly drive home was that I knew a lot of people, so how could I be lonely? It's a fair point and one which I found confusing as I worked out why I felt the way I did. How can I be lonely in that room? How can I be lonely with a large group of friends? I knew a lot of people and yet here I was tormented by a feeling that I was alone.

One morning as we walked on the beach I had a moment of clarity. It wouldn't matter if I knew 100,000 people, I would still be lonely because few if anyone really knew me at all. Or at least I felt that they didn't know me. The voice of loneliness that I heard over and over, my own mind speaking loneliness to me, was given voice because I felt unknown. My loneliness was not the condition of knowing very few people, it was the condition of being known by very few people. I was not alone, I felt lonely. That distinction felt important because it brought some hope. If there were people present in my life, then I could allow myself to be known by them. I could show the people that I already knew who I really was even though the thought felt terrifying. What if the real me actually was unlikeable.

As this book progresses you will understand the reasons why that felt terrifying. My understanding of myself was a tapestry of reality that had been spoiled by painful experiences, memories and lies about myself which I had believed. Overcoming low self-worth is a daily work and it is hard work. Overcoming a sense of inadequacy is a long-term project that is only progressed by working across our whole life and identity to restore false and broken ideas of self. The idea of letting someone into those spaces in my soul was scary enough to cause me to have sleepless nights and panic attacks.

When we stumble across moments of hope it is important to seize upon them when we have the chance. Hope is not the most common commodity and we should never take it for granted, for it is the most life-giving of things. Hope has the ability to raise our gaze to something beyond the pain. It strengthens our resolve and can give us something to live for. Never ignore it when you uncover it. Grab hold of it tightly.

In that moment of hope on the beach, began to question my sense of self. Why would I hide myself from people? What was I ashamed of? What made me fearful? What was the worst-case scenario in being known? If I was to answer these questions I needed help. So, after avoiding it for years, I booked in for some talking therapy for the first time in my life.

I will be honest. I had very low expectations. In light of every word, I have written above you will think the next sentence is ridiculous. I had always prided myself on being very self-aware, I considered myself to be someone who knew their own mind and understood why I acted the way I did. Why would I need to talk to a counsellor? Misplaced self-confidence is a hell of a drug! Yet, despite my lack of faith in its value, counselling was a conventional method for improving mental health so it seemed like a good thing to try.

I had never been more wrong in my expectations of something. Counselling was wonderful. Don't get me wrong, it was also exhausting and painful. Counselling moves from soothing and uplifting affirmation to a sense of having your skull torn open and someone poking their finger around in your psyche. It is both energising and arduous to have your mind attack and heal itself at the same time. I cannot recommend it you enough. Even if you feel perfectly healthy having an hour a week to just talk to a neutral person about the things that are on your mind is a healthy practice.

Very quickly I found myself spending much of those sessions naming and unpacking the things I was afraid of letting people know. I understood my fear of rejection was the strongest fear on the list. I was caught in a cycle of believing that if people really knew me that they would reject me so I would keep myself hidden in order to save myself from possible rejection that may never happen. In both pathways I'd designed in my head,, being rejected or keeping myself hidden, I was going to end up feeling lonely. This closed circle of damage had a strange comfort to it. I had tricked myself into believing that I was keeping myself safe. I was subconsciously telling myself that by choosing to be lonely, that was much less painful than being forced to be lonely by the rejection of others.

Our minds sometimes do that to us don't they? The negative and destructive patterns we choose are often in the guise of self-protection yet the results are the same. In my case, I was lonely either way, except rather than being made lonely I had chosen to be lonely. If I had been rejected and made lonely then I could find new people to build friendships with, there was a way out but I was choosing loneliness, the only escape from which was to choose to let myself be seen, really seen, warts (I don't have warts) and all. It was time to go public with my true self.

I am aware as I write this that the language of 'true self, going public and rejection' feels like dramatic language. Again, this is a trick that an anxious or depressed brain can play upon us. I will talk about this in the chapter on comparison. Often when we are suffering we tell ourselves that we are being dramatic. All that kind of thinking does is compound our struggle. Undermining our own feelings is a shield that protects our negative thinking. It insulates our damaging thoughts from examination. It keeps them intact and free from question. We will never overcome our pain if we cannot honestly see it for what it is. There is nothing dramatic in being honest with ourselves.

In therapy, I discovered that I was masking three main areas of my life and in doing so was keeping myself from ever really being known by anybody. There are three parts of my life which I continue to hide but much less so than I used to. The journey back to health is a long road that I will walk for the rest of my life. I came quickly to the realisation that I was hiding my beliefs about faith, I was hiding my fears and I was hiding my struggles.

I was turning up every week to this Christian group and when we discussed faith I felt like I was on a different page to many in the room. I chose to stay silent or to share a diluted version of my thoughts when I disagreed with someone because I was afraid of being banished to some theological exile.

I was silent about my fears because I felt I would look weak or faithless and therefore be rejected as some kind of lesser man or doubter.

I hid my struggles because I felt they were unworthy of attention. I felt that the things that I was afraid of, impending fatherhood, being unable to provide for my wife and child, my blood pressure killing me, my lack of any sense of career direction or that I was wasting my life, were irrational and invalid. If anyone knew these things they would think I was melodramatic or immature. I believed that anyone in their mid-thirties should have these things under control. By 35 you should have it all together, your ducks should be neatly in a row performing some kind of work-life balance conga.

Of course, the reality is that almost every adult I know, once I get to know them, feels like they are a bit of a blagger. I don't know anyone who doesn't feel like they are, at least in some way, out of their depth. I wait for the day when my 'I know what I'm doing' badge will arrive. Perhaps there is no destination in adulthood, it may just be a constant learning about who we are and how the world works, only to see ourselves and that world change as we learn. Perhaps we will never get a proper grip on things and the desire to grasp at life is causing us harm. Perhaps we should try to find a way to enjoy living and learn to accept that we will always feel that part of our world is out of our control. I think that could be a path to real liberation.

---

I began to open up. With my heart racing, I began to disagree. Disagreement, it turned out, was actually quite fun. People found my point of view at least a little bit interesting and I was not rejected. There were more heated moments of discussion, there were some baffled looks, there were times I was dismissive of other people's views and times that other people were dismissive of mine, but the discussions were life-giving. I was wrong about what would happen if I stopped hiding.

Staying silent and in essence choosing to be unknown, and therefore lonely, had been a huge mistake. There was room for my beliefs in the discussion, this seems so obvious now, but when I felt like the 'other' in the room that acceptance felt impossible. I shared my fears and felt seen. Others in the room shared some of those fears or had previously overcome them. I opened up about my struggles, people helped me to find perspective. I had removed my mask just a little and had begun to feel known for the first time in years. I was still often lonely, but rather than that being an unbroken drone in my life, drowning out my joy, it was now broken and punctuated by moments of feeling held and loved and known, truly known.

The voice of loneliness in my head was loud for a long time and on many occasions it still is. I had tried for years to silence or muffle it by meeting more people, building larger groups of friends, trying new hobbies to make memories with new people or by listening to other people's stories. The more I surrounded myself with people the more lonely I became because I was going about things backwards. I'm now convinced that, whilst knowing people is a cure for isolation, the only real cure for loneliness is allowing ourselves to be seen and known as we really are. The only cure for my loneliness was to take the risk of vulnerability. It was when I was sure people could see the real me, or at least a more real version of myself, and yet they still showed up in my life that that voice lowered in volume. My sense of loneliness became less intense as I deliberately let myself be known better. There are still days, of course, when I feel like I'm back to feeling invisible in a crowd of people but those times increasingly rarer. I am a little way down a much more healthy path.

What are the things that you hide from people? What are the parts of yourself that you keep from view and so stopping anyone from really getting to know you? Do you think you can overcome the fear of being known in order to defeat the sense of loneliness you feel?

My advice is this, make choices to fight back against that voice, but be kind to yourself. Start small with perhaps one person and let yourself experience both fear and acceptance at once in what is essentially a controlled environment. Be kind to yourself because the reality of this world is that there will be times when it doesn't go to plan and the person doesn't respond well. In those moments remind yourself that they, like you, live in a society that at times seems to be designed to destroy our mental health and self-worth. You never know what they are battling at that time and you can make allowances for that, but neither should you accept mistreatment, we are all worth much more than tolerating it. Take a risk in the next week, tell someone something you've wanted to say for a long time. You never know what might happen.

## 3. Appearance

I know they weren't making music for people like me, but One Direction did have some excellent tunes. However, in perhaps their biggest hit, they actually annoyed me because it was incredibly singable and yet laced with what is an incredibly negative message. In short, it's a nippy little ditty with lyrics that mean, 'You're insecure about how you look, that's what makes you beautiful.' I'm sure that wasn't the intention of the lyricist but it is there if you're a cynical reader like me. Anyway, you're not here for my strong opinions on boy bands.

Why do so many of us feel so awful about how we look? I am sure you instantly thought about magazines and adverts and movies in response to that question. I'm sure you thought about words like 'plus-sized' and 'size zero,' 'six-packs' and 'teeth whiteners.' The society we live in has created a mythology of idealised beauty that is haunting far too many of us, but rather than creating a pantheon of deities bearing superpowers, we have an ever-changing group of men and women who most closely fit the current notion of perfection. Men and women are caught in the comparison trap with Dwayne Johnson and Rihanna, Idris Elba and Margot Robbie all of whom will be comparing themselves to someone else. Whether it is marketing or a flaw in our nature I don't know, but all of us are comparing our looks to someone else's.

It seems that year on year the areas of our bodies that need to be perfected grows longer. Every time I go on social media these days I get adverts for a three-step product to stop my skin looking terrible. It has a beautiful young woman pawing at the face and neck of a slightly older man. 'Nothing is sexier than a man who cares of his skin,' she says with her puppy dog eyes looking straight down the camera. Apart from the clear lack of imagination in regards to what is sexy, this advert is telling me that the skin I have is wrong in some way. The skin that my genetic kaleidoscope has thrown around my organs, muscles and bones is not naturally good enough and in fact, is making beautiful young women like the one in the advert turn away in disgust. My skin, I am being told is unsexy, but if I smear it with three different creams in various shades of grey I will suddenly be incredibly desirable. Needless to say, I haven't invested. I have also not invested in the endless teeth whitening or hair restoring offers that beam their way from my phone to my brain every day. I've also accepted that I'm probably never going to have the right type of abs.

For women it seems that the list lengthens at an even faster rate and the acceptable requirements of the usual suspects on that list constantly change. Women's legs once deemed incredibly useful for things like walking or running, are now valued on their shape and the ideal shape changes based on who is topping the beauty charts at that moment. One year a woman's legs should be slender and sleek the next they are to be thick (thicc?) and curved. Trends spread across social media insisting a woman's body should have a thigh gap or bikini bridge. Women must also simultaneously have a torso the size of a small child whilst having breasts and bums that are large and curved but also able to defy gravity. I think they call this genetic balancing act being slim-thicc.

Women are told to paint their skin and dye their hair and wear false eyelashes. They must have eyebrows that are HD and on fleek but they dare not be too HD or they could be mocked endlessly as a meme. Their lips must be plump but not too plump. Ultimately, according to the internet, the majority of women look wrong. Your face as a woman is never going to be right. Paint it. Your body is wrong. Disguise it or change it by clever clothing, exercise or surgery. Look better, for that is your only value.

There was a moment when I became really aware of the reality of just how relentless the voices that undermine our self-perception are. I was watching Saturday evening television (think something vacuous but entertaining) and we reached an ad break. The first advert was for hair dye i.e. your hair is actually the wrong colour, if it was one of our chemically induced shades your life would be better, you'd get the partner of your dreams and you'd have way more fun. The second was for chocolate where a woman was having a bath with a 1 kg bar of the stuff. When she does it is alluring, when I do it I have depression. The third, from the same company as the hair dye was for a shampoo that won't fade the chemically induced dye of advert one. Then a car advert. The final advert of the break was for a conditioner, again by the same company. In essence, the message was, 'a woman's hair has to deal with so much these days. It is damaged by dyeing it and the shampoos you use to protect the dye are stripping it of its natural oils but our magical conditioner squeezed from the tear ducts of an angel and mixed with butterfly sweat will save the day.

In one short break in transmission of a prime time show, women were told their hair was the wrong colour and they should dye it. To keep their hair their new acceptable colour they should use the correct product and that dyeing it and using that product whilst completely essential meant they were destroying their hair, how stupid of them, they should use the conditioner to save it. 4 minutes of garbage designed to make money by making women feel like crap. It's pretty abhorrent.

The existence of a billion-pound industry based upon the setting of impossible standards of comparison and the subsequent exploitation of every day people's insecurities in light of those comparisons should be unacceptable to us all but for most of us, it is accepted with a shrug. The lie that anyone's body is wrong and can be fixed by chemicals or a knife should be met with disgust but the majority of us buy into it. How did we ever let this happen? How did we ever accept a message that drives people to mental distress based upon the shape of their body, their weight or their bone structure? We are surely better than this.

The second myth of our society is that mental suffering due to negative body image is limited to women. The research of the last decade has uncovered the increasing problem of negative body image amongst men, particularly younger men. Whilst men do not have to cope with the industrialised onslaught of negative messaging that women face, there is a growing issue amongst men. Terms like bigorexia have been coined to help describe the condition many men are dealing with. Their bodies are never right, they become addicted to working out and in some cases steroid use. Male use of plastic surgery is on the rise and men, as women have for years, are told that the natural state of their body is unacceptable.

The adverts that appear on my Facebook feed are anecdotal evidence of this. Perhaps the most fascinating advert recently is for a shaver especially design for male body and pubic hair. It's probably my own fault that it appeared, I made the mistake of clicking on an advert for a free trial of a shaving supplies subscription and it opened a whole can of worms. Having watched the advert for this magical short and curly shaver I have learned something I already knew. I have learned that men, when naturally prone to being at least partially hairy are deemed unacceptable by this company. They should have the build of a superman and the skin of a child. Their bodies should be covered in lumpy muscles that are in turn covered in soft smooth skin.

I can see the eye rolls of every woman reading that last paragraph. I know, I know. Women have lived with this body hair lie for years.

Women, girls in fact, since the day they grow their first body hair are told to shave it off, wax it off or epilate it off. Somewhere around 2002, the men of the world seemed to pass a law banning female public hair adding it to the list of leg hair and armpit hair. Why haven't women risen up and destroyed men yet? We deserve it.

It's much worse for women, but this society we accept and invest in is bad for all of our self-esteem.

I'm physically more or less average man. 6ish feet tall and a little bit more body fat than I should have. I have the recede of many men around 40 and I'm thinning on top as I thicken around the waist. My beard and the hair on my temples are well on their way to being white. Every time I look in the mirror I see the faces of my grandfathers gradually being revealed. Ageing is a trip. I'm a very normal-looking man. Yet, since the age of 14, had severe insecurities about how I look and 25 years later I sometimes feel the same way as I did back then, perhaps even worse.

The next few paragraphs should be read to the soundtrack of William Orbit's version of Adagio for Strings. It somehow captures the whole mood of this part of my life. I also realise the objective ridiculousness of the thoughts about my body that haunt me but objectivity is almost impossible for humans. We cannot remove ourselves from our experiences. Everything we think or feel is subjective and based on years of dealing with life.

Okay. Here goes. At this age of thirteen or fourteen, a sweet innocent boy with a mass of ginger curls on his head began to enter the dark and terrifying world of puberty. My voice began to drop an octave and hair appeared in surprising places. That hair unsurprisingly was also ginger. Of course,it was, I mean why wouldn't it be? Until that point in my life the colour of my hair had been an irrelevance but much to my surprise and horror it suddenly became very relevant.

3 days after my 14th birthday, on 27th February 1995, the BBC ran the first episode of three seasons of a sitcom called Game On. In short, a laddish comedy about 3 housemates, Matthew, Martin and Mandy, and their hilarious life in London. Well, the stand outline of that show became a stick with which my self-esteem was beaten. In almost every episode, Matthew, the cool one, would berate Martin, the uncool one, with at least one growl of 'Ginger Tosser!' Cue canned laughter,

Before I'd made it to school assembly at 9 am on 28th February 1995, at least 7 people, none of whom I actually knew had shouted 'ginger tosser' at me. Cue real laughter. I'd not seen the show and had no idea why this was happening. By the end of March, this had become a daily ritual. My body was changing, I had normal, hormone-induced teenage angst and now had the consistent mockery of my peers to deal with.

It didn't stop at 'ginger tosser' either. Teenagers are as creative in their teasing as they are naive about its consequences. Here is a concise list of excellent banter I was on the receiving end of:

Ginger pubes (This was basic biology)

Gingaling (Clever rhyming)

Ginger Wanker (I mean. It wasn't untrue. I was 14 years old)

Ginge Minge (Perhaps a further biology lesson was required for the genius who came up with this one)

Mandarin Pubes (Someone had read the Dulux colour chart)

Fanta pants (This insult is sponsored by the Coca-Cola company)

I mostly laughed it off and did what a lot of kids do, I attempted to limit its impact by getting the joke in first. I found myself calling myself those things when people were joking around in the hope I'd feel less pain of feeling singled out. It didn't work.

In fact, it led to the most thought-through joke of them all. The Anti-Ginger Front. My friends, and to be clear they had no idea it was hurting me at all because I laughed along, created an imaginary movement which called for such things as Ginger Segregation in the Classroom, Gingers to be required to clean any chair and desk after use and to have all gingers neutered in order to no longer pollute the gene pool. The AGF came with photocopied posters and slogans written on chalkboards in lessons and jokes at my expense. 'Yeah but you're ginger,' was a common response to most of what I said. A lot of effort to go to, I admire their commitment to laughter.

I laughed along and in retrospect realise that nobody was consciously trying to humiliate me, or at least I hope they weren't. By the lack of reaction I had they would have assumed I was fine and untouched by the jokes but I wasn't. I was crying at home. I remember asking God to make my hair brown (God has since responded later in life with a lot of my hair falling out and turning white). I really wanted it to stop. I changed how I behaved in certain situations in order to avoid the comments. I'd wear a beanie at rugby training as 'ginger's ball' very quickly moved to 'ginger balls.' I changed for swimming hidden under a towel. I hated my hair and the curse that puberty and the BBC had brought to my body. Nobody knew how miserable I was.

I realise that to an adult that story is quite ridiculous. I realise that to an adult that kind of teasing would be shrugged off but as a child becoming an adult through the terror of being a teenager it left a mark. The worst thing is that the effects still remain. I still find myself aware of my hair colour. I still change under a towel for fear of someone catching a glimpse of something and yelling out 'Fanta pants.' I'm on the verge of turning 40 and the jokes still hurt. Our painful memories are the hardest to forget.

Add into that mix the joy that, in the words of Paul Simon, I'm 'soft in the middle now,' and I could easily begin to hate how I look. I've managed to evade this so far by changing how I understand what my body is for.

I'm thankful for movements like I Weigh[2], spearheaded by the wonderful Jameela Jamil. The message is that the weight of who you are, your character and achievements, is much more important than the number of pounds the needle on the bathroom scales hits. That's so wonderfully true; my value is never measured by the weight or appearance of my body. Nor is yours.

---

[2] https://iweighcommunity.com

I've also begun to value my body for what it can do and not for how it looks. My body can take me to beautiful places. My body can taste red wine and blue cheese. My body can hug my children and kiss my wife. My body can create music and splash in the sea. My body provides me with every good experience in my life. I must choose to keep it healthy because I value those experiences and want to live for a long time.

My body is no more or less valuable because my hair is ginger or my waist is a few more inches around than it once was . My body is valuable because I live in it and it can take me anywhere I choose to go and give me the experiences I want to have.

Your body is no more or less valuable because it's old or young. Your body is no more or less valuable because you are disabled or abled. Your body is no more or less valuable because you are cis or transgender. Your body is no more or less valuable because of your skin tone or hair colour. Your body is no more or less valuable because you are heavy or light, thick or thin. The size of your breasts or penis or bum or biceps will never change your value. They mark out your worth no more than the shape of your elbow does. You are valuable because you are, and your body is valuable because you are in it. It is not wrong. You are not wrong. It is yours.

What can your body do? What are you thankful for being able to achieve with your body? What memories have you made with your body? Celebrate what your body had enabled you do? How your body looked when you did these good things wasn't in all likelihood that relevant.

Our bodies are wonders. Our bodies are as beautiful as they are different. When we can celebrate them we can begin to lower the volume of the voices that tell us we look the wrong way. Celebrate yourself. Your body has brought many joys to the world. You deserve the praise.

Your body might be able to run fast and climb high. It might be able to read books and write songs. Your body may have carried you through racism, homophobia, misogyny or ableism. Your body may have continued to transport you through a world that was not designed for someone with your condition and you have overcome so much.l with it. Your body might have beaten cancer. Your body might have carried children, and delivered them to the world. Your body is not wrong. There is no standard.

Your body will bear scars and bruises of the life you've lived but you are still here, your heart is beating and your lungs are breathing. Celebrate every day you get to live in it. You are not wrong. You just are and the way you are is not just worth acceptance it is worth praising and honouring. Choose to delight in yourself. You're excellent.

## 4. Comparison

Theodore Roosevelt is much more quotable that some US Presidents I can think of. One quote that is often attributed to him is the deeply wise, 'comparison is the thief of joy.' It's hard to dream up a phrase that more accurately describes the damage comparison does to our sense of who we are, it literally steals the joy from our existence. Yet, despite this being true we are all addicted to comparison.

Of course, comparison is drilled into us from an early age. Our childhoods are filled with comparisons, both innocent and sinister, that teach us to look around us and notice where we stand in the crowd. As 4-year-olds, we line up against the wall from tallest to shortest to get chosen for a game. We are graded into bands of academic and creative performance; I'm a C grade, she is an A. We compare our school bags and hairstyles and trainers as kids and in our heads, grade the owners of those objects as better or worse than ourselves.

As adults we compare bank balances, house sizes, car models. We compare lifestyles and holidays. We compare lives with children or lives childfree. We compare job titles and achievements. We compare everything. We are forger those 4-year-olds finding their place against the wall hoping not to be the smallest boy or girl in class. We never seem to grow out of comparison even though it makes us all sad.

A 2015 study[3] by researchers Nanyang Technological University, Singapore, and Bradley University and the University of Missouri in the United States found that, after studying the effects of Facebook use on 700 US college students. The study found that 'Facebook envy,' led to increased feelings of jealousy and dissatisfaction which in turn exacerbated or led to feelings and symptoms of depression. Comparison was young adults miserable when they should have been enjoying their first steps into the world.

As a teenager, I really wanted a pair of what are now known as Nike Air Max 1s. They were at that time unaffordable for my hard-working parents and I got a pair of perfectly excellent Nike Air Pegasus. A few

[3] https://doi.org/10.1016/j.chb.2014.10.053

school friends had Air Max 1s and I was jealous. I find it strange that 25 years later I still regularly look at Air Max 1s and consider buying them 1 as if it will somehow make a difference to that teenage version of me. Comparison doesn't just attack our joy in the moment, it can keep attacking us for years.

Today I get caught in much less trivial comparisons, almost always in the privacy of my own head. I compare how well I provide for my children. I compare my children's behaviour. I compare how clever they are. I compare my car and home. I compare how popular I feel. I compare how successful I feel in my career and how much my salary is. I compare how I look. I compare how much sex I have or don't have. I compare my holidays and my clothes. The temptation to compare is constant and it is very rare that I end up on the good side of the comparison. More often than not, I feel like I'm less than the one with whom I contrast my existence.

Of course, some level comparison is a natural part of being human but the incessant comparison we are addicted to is turbocharged by marketing and social media posts. Our eyes and therefore our minds are constantly fed images and ideas to compare ourselves to. So much of our world is rated into top ten lists and best sellers and our views of each other are at risk being no different. We like and share and retweet the details of one another's lives, grading each other's existence in a silent popularity contest that nobody ever wins. I'm pretty sure that it's declared war on our self-worth.

Comparison, however, doesn't only steal joy from us, it can also rob us of the ability to receive help. Perhaps the last significantly damaging moments of comparison in my life were the times when I needed help, but, in comparing my suffering to others, I deemed my problems insignificant. We tell ourselves that things aren't that bad or that others have it much worse and in essence, lower our own value to the point of being unworthy of help.

There will be people reading this now who are suffering from mental health struggles, relationship difficulties, physical struggles and financial problems who have looked around and decided someone else's problems were worse. These people, who deserve and need help and support, have never asked for it because comparison has told them the lie that their pain is not worth healing. They have been trapped by thoughts that tell them it could be worse, so they should just accept and find a way to survive how bad things are now. Comparison is also the thief of freedom, restoration and healing.

'He verbally abuses me but has never hit me, it's not that bad.'

'She controls me and makes me miserable but at least she is faithful.'

'It's only missing one meal. So many have it much worse.'

'I've nothing to be sad about. I should just pull myself together.'

These are the lies that comparison tells us; that we need to soldier on because someone else has overcome something that we deem to be more difficult. One of the lessons I've found it hardest to learn is that whilst the causes of our pain are different, our experiences of pain are equally real. Suffering is suffering and every soul that experiences it is worth helping to escape from or manage that suffering. My suffering is no less real to me because I've deemed the cause of it to be trivial in comparison to yours.

The verbal abuse you suffer is no less real because you know others suffer physical abuse. Your depression is no less real because you do not have suicidal ideation. Your poverty is no less real because someone else has less than you. Your pain is real. Your suffering is real. Your fear is real. You deserve to be free of it if that is possible. Comparison tells us to suffer in silence but we are all worth more than our silence.

I'm convinced that gratitude is the antidote for comparison. Comparison can poison every part of our lives, and gratitude can neutralise that poison. Joy is one of the most powerful things on earth and yet we have designed a society that kills it. Gratitude can bring it back to life.

Being grateful for my health overcame my need to compare my body to other more chiselled men. Being grateful for my well-paid job overcame my need to compare my success to other more wealthy people. Being grateful for the love in my home overcame my need to compare my lifestyle to anyone else's.

It wasn't an easy transition. I had to discipline myself to speak words of gratitude out loud. I don't think that our words have some mystical power to speak things into existence but I do think vocalising things forces us to hear the truths we are choosing to hold. I believe the same about writing those truths down. Reading our own words can bring transformation that just having the very same thoughts does not.

In working hard to speak and write gratitude for my life I found that my desire to compare diminished. I found that being grateful for the small and large details of my life causes me to lose interest in where those details fell on some made-up value scale when compared to the details of other lives. It is liberating. I've a long way to go but the increased sense of freedom is intoxicating. Joy is a delight.

If I could recommend one practice to you in overcoming comparison, it is to set time aside each day to actively focus on being thankful for your life. I'm a person of faith, so it often takes the form of a prayer of thankfulness for me, but it is no less relevant a practice to an atheist or agnostic. Create a daily practice of giving thanks for what you have, what you've achieved, for the people in your life and for the memories you've made. Speak those words of thanks out loud or write them in a journal. Be thankful for the little moments, the oat milk flat white and the smile of a stranger. Be thankful for the big things too, the promotion and the marriage, the home and the first date.

The only path that leads to a joyful existence is the path of gratitude. Discontent will destroy us in the end. That road leads to misery. Nothing will ever be good enough. Real joy is in the contentment with what we have now, for if we receive more it will be a celebration on top of already existing joy. A comparison driven need for more is insatiable, there is always more to covet. Where our lives are good we must call them good.

Choose as best you can to love your life, choose to love it as it is now and for the parts of your life which you can't love because you are unsafe or being hurt then get help to get out of those situations. Escape the relationship that is abusing you. Get therapy and medication for your troubled mind. Apply for jobs and study for a new career path if you hate your job. Ask for help if your finances are struggling to support your life.

I'm convinced this is the only way to discover joy and peace in our lives; to love what we can about our life and to seek help to escape the troubles. We are worth it. We are all worth celebrating and we are all worth helping. I'm learning to believe this, I hope you can believe it too.

## 5. Calling

Some people age like a fine wine, some like a rotten egg, either way, are all getting older. I'm 39 years old and since my 35th birthday, become more aware of my mortality than I had in the previous years of my life. This thought came as a real surprise to me, for in real terms, I'm not very old, I've plenty of decades left to live, my body is reasonably healthy and life is good. Yet, that year was the year that a quiet little voice in my head started talking about the fact that I'm getting older.

Now don't get me wrong, it isn't that I lived in some fantasy land where I still felt 21, that's not what I mean at all. That youthful sense of being indestructible was long gone. I've had enough near misses with traffic to knock that out of me. I've long put to bed the reckless abandon of my early 20s, where taking stupid risks was just part of life. I'm not talking about a sense of impending death or a sense of the fragility of life. This is something different.

You see, the voice in my head didn't point to my consistently sore knee or my grey beard and remind me that I was getting older. The voice in my head, let's be clear, my own thoughts, ran over the same phrases every time it raised its voice.

'You're running out of time. It's too late. You'll never do the things you dreamt of now.'

I've never been much into regular ambition or status. I don't dream of a big house and a Tesla. I don't know why those things have just never given me much of a buzz. I'm more drawn to the adventure of building communities and seeing the legacy of those communities lived out in the lives of those who were part of them. The few ambitions that I've ever had have been about building things that individual people remember, not because they were big, flashy or famous things, but because, for those people, they helped them in some way at some precise time. The reality is, I tell myself, often against the evidence, that I've not been pursuing those ideas for a very long time.

I know that I'm being vague about my dreams and ambitions, but that is because it's really hard to describe them. It is something that would be hard to express to you but when it is happening, I recognise it and I haven't seen it in years. It is the idea that I've not been seeing it in years that allows that phrase to cause me harm. That voice in my head tells me that I'm wasting my time doing all of the things I'm doing now and I'm running out of time to do the thing I'm supposed to do.

Let's take a moment to unpack that last sentence. 'What I'm supposed to do?' Really? The older I get the less I actually believe that any of us are here to perform specific jobs that are uniquely assigned to us by some force in the universe. I don't think I believe that 'everything has a purpose' and in fact, I think searching for a purpose in many of the painful things that happen to us causes us to increase the damage caused by traumas we experience.

There was a time, however, when I believed that kind of thing with all my heart. I was sure I was put on earth with a job to do, like some kind of ginger Superman with a much less impressive set of skills. I spent a decade of my life in a stream of Christianity in which this was a constant conversation. Books and talks and conferences focussed on knowing your calling and purpose in life. That idea sank deep into my psyche and it is not easily uprooted. All these years later I am much more convinced that we make the best go of what we happen to have in life and if there is any call, it is to love people, serve people, be kind and to leave the world better than we found it. That on its own is a big enough job.

It would be a mistake to think that it is only people of faith who get drawn into this way of thinking. We spend our days immersed in stories that tell us the same thing. Every movie is played out along a path of destiny that leads the characters to the end of their tale. Romance is tied up with the language of 'soul mates' and 'meant to be.' Whether it is divine calling, destiny or whether it is written in the stars, we are surrounded by messaging that tells us there are things that are meant to happen and we must be careful not to miss them.

Ultimately, that is because this messaging sells. It sells because so many of us are afraid that we are not fulfilling our potential. It sells because so many of us spend our days doing things that are many miles removed from what we hoped for as children. It sells because many of us have unrequited feelings for someone, or have lost 'the one.' It sells because we are afraid of living what we imagine to be sorry little lives that will be forgotten within a few years of our deaths. It sells because we feel insignificant.

Believing in destiny and calling can cushion us from some of that pain. If it is our destiny, then one day we will be lifted from the job we hate and cast into the adventure we dream of. If it is our calling, we will one day find ourselves on the metaphorical stage we've felt we were made for. If these ideas are true, then even the messes we have made can be redeemed, and in some way serve to make us even better at that one thing we are made for. The idea of destiny is a comfort in a world that is hard, it gives us hope that one day we might get out of the place we are in, and be in that place that we imagine to be much better.

I get it, I really do. I lived it for years and years. When I was at my lowest ebb the idea that this was somehow working me towards my calling got me up in the morning. When I was doing jobs that I hated I told myself that it would be only a short time before 'it' happened. Life is hard and the thought of it being filled with direction can feel like a warm hand on a cold night. I get it, but I think that if I embraced that idea again it would end up ruining my life.

For those who believe in destiny or calling who also believe that they are living their destiny and calling it is a great idea, but for those who feel lost or dissatisfied that belief is a weight around their necks that will soon drag them down. The idea that there is something else better to come can do two things to a person. It can cause them to stop. wait and stagnate in expectation of the big thing to happen, or they can grow to hate the life they are living now, as their dissatisfaction grows with life in the 'place they are not meant to be'.

I've met people in both of those situations and I've been the person in both of those situations. I've been the person who waits for a sudden event that suddenly changes everything. I've sat with friends who believe their destiny to be just around the corner and spend years of their life waiting as time passes by, time in which they could have been working towards something or building joy and experiences into their life. They just seemed to hit pause on everything except waiting. They existed when they could have been thriving. I've been one of those people.

I've also met people who fall deep into depression because they deeply believe the life they are living is not the life they are supposed to live. They feel that there is something more for them, something better and that thought begins to invade every experience and relationship they have. Moments that should be sweet become bittered by never being good enough because they aren't 'the thing.' If we live long enough in that place the idea that happiness and fulfilment are only available in the imagined situation quickly kills the joy of every real situation we are in.

I've had periods of time when I've been haunted by this idea that I'd missed the boat, that I wasn't fulfilling my calling or that I was in the wrong place. It is something I have had to battle regularly because that thought is extremely bad for me and it finds its root in my once long-held idea of calling. So my idea of calling had to go. It is bad for me because I became lethargic in everything I did that I didn't connect to my calling. It is bad for me because I began to miss the joys of the moment. It is bad for me because it let resentment leak into my marriage and my relationships with my children. It caused me to jump from job to job looking for the one that was closest to 'the dream.' I was never going to be satisfied. If I didn't let go of my idea of calling it was going to ruin my life. I caught onto the problem early enough but I dread to think where it would have led me if I had not.

The idea that there is a life that I will one day reach that is more suited to us than the one I live now has the power to switch off our ability to live in the present. The idea that we are moving towards somewhere special makes where we are now less special. Living in some future utopia turns the present into nothing more than a trial to survive until we reach the life that we really want. When we are striving for an imagined destination we miss the real beauty of where we are now. We have to learn to live in the moment we are in and allow the future to be what it will be.

I have no advice on how to do it. I just actively tell myself to enjoy the moment. I am deliberately thankful for the people in my life and the place I am now. I am grateful for my wife and our boys. I am grateful for my friends. This life I am living in now is wonderful. If there is better than this on the way, so be it, I'll embrace and enjoy it but I will no longer allow the idea that there is something better coming along to sully and denigrate the wonder of the life I live now. It isn't easy, I feel like I'm constantly removing the idea from my thoughts, but the more I work at it the easier it gets.

May you also find a way to be fully present where you are. May you learn to embrace today with all of its beauty. May you hold your dreams lightly and your present tightly. May you never miss the beauty of the day you are in by throwing it under the shadow of an imagined future.

## 6. Significance.

Cold air. The lasting memory of that moment is how cold the air felt agonist my face. I walked through the door, lilac on the inside, black on the outside and felt cold air on my face and then jumped slightly as the door banged shut behind me. I could feel that the back of my shirt was clung to my back as the stress sweat had pulled it close to my skin. The cold air was a relief. I remember looking up at the darkened, outside of the Rose Window of York Minster and said out loud, 'what now?'

If I wanted to, I could stand in that same spot in the centre of York and relive that moment from a Saturday morning almost a decade ago. It would feel as fresh and recent as if it happened this morning. On that day I was sure a story in which I would find my greatness had come to an end. I'd spent every day of my life since the age of 16 reading, learning and working towards one thing. I had plans, long term plans, for how my life would look. I had books and folders filled with notes and ideas. I had poured my heart and soul into other people until I felt empty. It had been a long time passed and a lot of miles travelled in those 15 years and I could finally see what I'd been building taking shape. Then it fell apart. That door closing behind me as I walked alone into the cold morning air knocked the final brick to the ground. It was over.

The dream I lost? Well, it seems strange now to think that it had consumed my whole being for a decade and a half, but it was to build a community of faith in which anyone could thrive and invest their passion. It was to lead a community in which people found their voice and their goodness and then shared both with the world. I'd waited a long time and it was finally there. It was small and it was chaotic at times but it was so life-giving and fulfilling. It had cost me a lot to build and then it was gone.

Just as my dream materialised, my home life fell apart and quickly afterwards meetings were organised, people, some of whom I barely knew, gave their opinions on my state of mind. Advice flooded in as quickly as rumours flooded out. Within a week of my marriage beginning to end, my resignation was requested and within a weekend it was given; a letter laid on a desk, stairs descended and a door, lilac on the inside and black on the outside, closed shut behind me. Cold air.

I've had a decent share of pain in life, many have suffered more, many have suffered less, but there has been no single day in which I felt more alone in the world than on that one. I felt lost and forgotten. I felt a level of emotional exhaustion and hopelessness that as so intense it made my body ache. I had no idea what I could possibly do next. 'What now?' I asked the cold air. Silence.

I had given every day of my adult life to pursuing something that in 10 days had evaporated into the air and I felt as if a huge chunk of my identity had gone with it. I felt that the one thing that made me anywhere close to great in anyone's eyes was gone. The one thing that I had ever felt good at was taken from me. If I was honest felt like I was done. I was over.

I talked about this moment and the feelings wrapped up with my memory of it when I was in counselling, and it is clear that I had an unhealthy relationship with that dream of mine. I had allowed it to define me, to become a central part of who I am. The reality is that I was never what I did, what I did was always an outworking of who I am. I had allowed things to get the wrong way round, and that had exponentially amplified the trauma I was already experiencing.

All these years later and I haven't ever, until now, written down the impact that experience had on my life. As we edge towards ten years since it happened, I am beginning to realise that, although deeply scarring, that the path I was forced onto by those events is leading me to a place of freedom from the voice that haunts me the most. That voice that tells me that I need a legacy, that I need greatness and that I need significance. It also tells me to look for those things in all the wrong places. In therapy, I became aware that the wound I felt the deepest from those ten days a decade ago was the idea that I had lost my chance at a legacy and instead had been forced into insignificance.

I realise these are dramatic words that would be much better placed in the biography of a general or politician than in the story of a young man leading a very small church community. I am aware that this language seems misplaced, but whether deluded or not, that is what I felt was happening. The one thing that I was building that I believed would outlast me was gone. The one thing that made me feel consequential was no more.

We live in a society which idolises fame. Our movies are filled with men and women who seize their moment and change the world. We have built machines that keep us connected, 24 hours a day, to the lives, or the published lives at least, of the people we deem to be most significant to the planet. We post 280 character thoughts online and check back to see how many people deemed our words worth a click that took them a fraction of a second to do. We celebrate when our Instagram followers hit 50, 500 or 1000 or more. The message is that visibility is to be pursued, for in being recognisable we achieve significance. Of course,all of this kind of behaviour predates social media but social media has sent it into hyperdrive and that is no good thing.

The promise that we are seeking through our online lives is, of course, a lie. Deep down we all know that, but I and many others have swallowed that lie right up and lived accordingly. Living in the shadow of that false promise has caused me significant emotional harm. Living life in pursuit of visibility, greatness or significance has made me ill. It has kept we awake at night. It has caused me panic attacks. It has sent me into depression. It has made me ill because the hunger for significance in the recognition of others will never be satisfied. The need to leave a legacy will never be met because it is impossible to know ahead of time what we will be remembered for or whether we will be remembered at all. Pursuing that knowledge is a fool's errand that will only end in heartache. Yet that voice in my head kept telling me to chase it.

-----

I watched the Disney+ recording of Hamilton for the first time tonight. The song that is quoted at the top of this chapter brought me to tears. I've listened to the soundtrack of Hamilton many times. I have heard this song before but it wasn't until watching it play out on my television that I really felt its truth. Eliza Hamilton sings it to her husband, the protagonist of the show, Alexander. He has just been sent home from the field office of George Washington in disgrace; he had thrown away his shot at greatness. His chance at significance was gone. He returned to his wife, who reveals she is pregnant, and then sings a song begging her husband to see that there was no need for a legacy or money, but that being loved by her and their son could be enough. To them, he was everything. Could they be that for him?

My mind quickly left the year 1778 and was taken to the daily-repeated scene of our family breakfast at my own kitchen table. Those words cut deep into that part of me that, in spite of counselling, still looks for recognition, greatness and significance in all the wrong places. For that same voice that tells me to strive and search for those three things, is also telling me that the actual three greatest things in my life are not enough for me. The idea that there is some greater significance to be found hides within its terms that the devotion of the woman who loves me more than I could ever ask, and of the two boys whose faces light up when they see me, is not enough.

As Philippa Soo sang those words, I heard them in the voice of my wife, for she has said them to my unlistening ears before.

'We don't need to be rich, Dave. We don't need some sort of legacy. We can be enough.'

If I could rewind my life, I would search for the moment that I first caught the idea that significance was found in my achievements and I would try to change my course. I will never find significance in what I achieve because there will always be more to achieve and more again after that. I will never be satisfied. It is a thirst that is unquenchable.

In about 6 hours time, I will be awoken by a 2-year-old banging on his door for my attention. I will be jumped on by a 5-year-old who has a habit of landing his knees into tender places as he leaps onto our bed. I will feel a hand on my shoulder from the other side of that same bed, as a slumber laden voice greets me into the day. I will spend wonderful moments laughing at the terrible jokes and puns of my favourite person, as she tries to bring little sparks of joy into my day. I will be asked questions about science and maths and trees and music by a curious little mind. I will get slobbery kisses from the most affection boy I've ever met. In the eyes of the people, love the most and would do anything for, I have great significance. I am central to their world. I don't have to impress them. I don't have to do anything at all to be significant to them. I just need to show up.

I have a lot of work to do to silence the voice that tells me that I'm not enough because I have not done enough of worth. I am more aware tonight than ever that I will not be the one who silences that voice, it will be silenced by the love of those who care for me for whom I will always be significant. Could that be enough? I really think it could be.

## A Moment of Pause 1 - Medication

'Crazy pills.'

When someone sees me taking my daily anxiety medication and asks me what they are for that is my reply. I don't know if it is the fact that I am from the island of Ireland, or if it is some deeper dysfunction, but this reply is typical of my propensity to self-deprecate. In my head, these kind of comments are an attempt at diffusing the awkwardness of the situation by making the focus of the conversation my blunt answer rather than the fact that I have to take medication to stop my own brain from attacking me.

The truth is, that even though I live my anxiety in a very public way, I still have some stock in the idea that needing medication for a mental health condition is shameful. That, of course, is a lie. If taking a paracetamol for a headache is fine, then taking a selective serotonin reuptake inhibitor to stop me having panic attacks whilst driving in traffic is also fine. When we are ill, we treat the illness. Sometimes that requires a pill.

I am writing this short section because I am convinced that many people I know should consider being on medication for their mental health, but either through stigma or fear of the unknown impact it might have upon them, they have avoided the conversation with their doctor. I believe that the only way to undermine a stigma and fear is by truth-telling. So I will give you the warts and all low-down on my experience with 'meds.'

Firstly, I should have been on these pills years ago. They have made an incredible difference in my life. Since I have been taking one pill a day, I am more stable, settled, positive and calm than I had been in perhaps 15 years. If I can describe the way these pills have affected my day to day life, I would way that the lowest lows of sadness and the highest highs of chaotic anxiety have been shaved off. It is as if the range of emotions I experience, the boundaries of which had reached into destructive spaces, has been narrowed between much healthier boundaries. My body is physically less tense and my thinking is much more clear. That's the positive side and if your doctor recommends you take medication for your mental health, seriously consider taking their advice. My experience is that it has almost exclusively been a good thing for me.

I take one pill a day of a medication called Citalopram. I have been taking it for just under 18 months. I take it with breakfast every day except on the days I forget to. If I forget one day, I don't notice any ill effect. That takes some pressure off. I have regular reviews with my GP about how I am doing with the medication and whether they think I am on the right dosage or not. It is like taking any other medication in that regard.

When I first started taking the drug it had three negative effects which lasted about 3 weeks. These may not be universal, I am not a doctor or pharmacist so wouldn't claim to speak with authority about side-effects, but these were my experiences.. All three of these side-effects were extremely manageable and did not impact hugely upon my day-to-day. They also seemed to ease very quickly as my body got used to the medication.

The first side-effect was that I was prone to suddenly overheating. I am unsure why this was but 'the sweats' were very sudden and very real. They were especially bad in bed at night. I drank more water and wore lighter clothing. Within a month it stopped happening. The second effect I noticed was that for the first few weeks of taking the medication my hands shook slightly. I was the only person who noticed, and it passed within 21 days. It may not have been connected to the medication but it coincided with starting taking the pills.

The final effect was drowsiness. At about 2:30 pm every day I wanted to nap. There were days when I first started my medication that I felt I was going to fall asleep on my laptop as I worked. Again, as with the other three early effects of the medication, this seemed to normalise again within a few weeks.

I write this because the stories we hear about the impacts mental health medication has on people rarely include stories like mine. There were initial effects, they were not debilitating. Of course, for some people on some higher dosages, or on different medication the effects might be vastly different in symptom or impact, but for me, the impact was very manageable.

I did not put on weight. I did not lose weight. I stayed the same, 102 kg, give or take the weight of a large pizza or pint.

The only long term impact that taking medication has had on me is that at times it is close to impossible, or impossible to orgasm. I'm sorry for being so blunt, but I think honesty about what you might expect is important in braking a stigma.

Almost unlimited sexual stamina? The Holy Grail right? Wrong. It has been at times incredibly frustrating to the point of causing almost as much anxiety than my initial anxiety condition. However, if I had to trade off the way I felt every day before taking the pills off against the moments of frustration the pills have caused in our bedroom, there is no comparison. I would choose to take the pills every time.

Again, I am only telling my story here, and this one lasting side-effect may not happen to everyone, for some it might be worse, for some it might be better, that is for a GP to advise on, but I share it because of people know what they might experience they are more equipped to seek help.

If you have recognised that you are unwell I cannot recommend a conversation with a GP highly enough. I had my conversation with my GP because I reached a point where I was not coping at all. I knew I should have had it much earlier. It came to the point where I had two panic attacks whilst at work. The reasons I didn't go to the doctor were fear of the unknown, fear that the drug would remove my personality and that I didn't want the stigma of taking 'crazy pills.' Each of those were genuine and legitimate fears but were based on things that were worth overcoming or lies.

Please talk to your GP. You are worth so much more than spending your days feeling miserable. You deserve to be helped. You deserve to recover. You deserve to be free is your pain.

I'm happy to answer any question about my experience with medication. Send me a message on twitter @davemagill and we can talk.

## 7.   Shame

Have you ever watched those videos on youtube where they place objects from everyday life underneath an hydraulic press and slowly add pressure until they snap, buckle, or explode from the weight on them? If you haven't, I recommend that you search them out. There is something strangely calming about watching a bottle slow-motion-shattering into minute pieces, or a basketball bouncing back into shape once the pressure is released.

There is one video I watched in which a 6-inch copper pipe, like the one a plumber might run to your radiator, is put vertically under the press. As the press comes down, the pipe slowly folds into perfectly symmetrical ripples, as if there is some sentience within it that tells it how to react to the load. In ten seconds the structure of the pipe changes completely from a smooth and useful tube of copper to a short and crumpled lump of the orange metal.

I can think of numerous moments in my life for which that collapsing copper pipe is a perfect analogy. I can easily bring to mind words spoken to me, or situations I was in that made me feel like that pipe. One moment I am stood tall and the next I am crumpling down under the weight of what has just happened; my self-esteem being pressed flat by the shame that suddenly hung around my shoulders.

There are fewer things that are more toxic than shame. Unchecked shame has the ability to ruin someone's entire life. Moments of shame can cause us to retreat into the darkness of whatever corner we can hide in. It can force us to let go of the things we have worked for, the people we love and the hope that we've worked hard to muster. One moment of shame, if left to fester can cast a long shadow over our lives and stop us from enjoying the beauty that is all around us.

My earliest memory of feeling ashamed feels like such a trivial thing, yet I can send myself back 33 years to experience it again as if it had just happened. It amazes me that a moment in time from my childhood can still cause me to feel the same emotions that I felt back then.

I can remember that it was raining and the hood of my coat was up as I stood in the corner of the school playground with two other 6-year-old boys. One of the boys invited the other to their birthday party and turned to me and said, 'you can't come, only the good people can come.' I can so clearly remember looking down to my feet and seeing the drops of rain on my black leather school shoes as that strange mix of a chill on my neck and heat in my cheeks rushed over me. I can remember feeling confused because it was the first time I was aware of being rejected and shamed by another person. I remember asking myself why I wasn't good. What was wrong with me?

It is so strange to think that a moment of school playground pettiness can still bring a chill to my neck.I don't tell you that story so that you feel sorry for 6-year-old me. As I said, this event is so small in the grand scheme of my life, I am obviously fine about it now. I share that story to draw attention to the fact that remembering that experience can still have an effect on me. I share this story because it illustrates that the shame we feel throughout our lives can stay with us for a long time. I share it because I think we all have a long list of moments like that in our lives that stretch back into our childhood and if we give them too much space in our heads, they can begin to take over and wreak havoc.

I can leaf back through my memories and pull out more moments like this. My first disastrous kiss. My first break up. Numerous rejections and slights. The friends who failed to stand by me when I needed them. The wrong clothes. The people who verbally abused me. The time someone through a hot kettle at me in anger. The wrong accent. The man who I respected who told teenage me that I didn't have what it takes to do the things that I wanted most to pursue. The moment I opened a decree absolute and the weight of what had happened in my past relationship hit me hard. Each of these memories carries with them that same chill on my neck and that same heat on my face; the outward symptoms of shame.

I made the mistake of allowing myself to believe that those experiences were connected. I made the mistake of believing that there was some link between the shame I felt as an uninvited 6-year-old and being told I didn't have what it takes as an adult. I allowed myself to take isolated incidents in my life and write them as some sort of narrative about who I was and what value I held. I allowed feelings of shame in unconnected moments to become a gathered diary of events that told me I should be ashamed, I was not good enough, I deserved to be treated badly and that these moments were all the evidence I needed that this was true. That story very quickly became incredibly destructive and it is taking a lot of time to stop believing it.

The belief that those isolated, painful moments are connected has played out in my work life and in my personal life. When my belief in that story has been strong, it plays out in my inability to push myself forward for anything at all. When the story is read aloud in my brain, it causes me to expect rejection, to undermine myself constantly and to self-sabotage. My self-penned story of shame has stopped me applying for jobs, ruined friendships and caused me to walk away from things I've loved doing. It has told me I will never belong, and I will never amount to the things I hope to become. Shame is a liar and a thief. I know, because I drank deep from its well and it poisoned me when I did.

Shame is what happens when moments in which we felt embarrassed are erroneously gathered together to form a complex narrative that tells that we are inadequate. That feeling of inadequacy will continually oppress us if we don't find a way to break the false connections in our minds. If my experience is anything to go by, this is a long and hard work that will involve self-reflection and, in my opinion, talking with a good therapist.

My wife, who is the person who has had to deal with me at my lowest ebbs, has a question she asks when she sees that a sense of inadequacy is rising up within me. A typical situation is that I've written some blog or article and am talking myself out of letting anyone read it. Alternatively, I'm suggesting I am not good enough to put my name forward for a job or task. In short, the thoughts of shame in my head have found a voice, my voice, and I am talking myself down and out of anything good that might come my way. She asks, 'What would you say to Andy or Ellie or Paul if they said what you just said about yourself, about themselves?' Cue a glint in her eye that is both comforting and infuriating because I know she is right.

Sheepishly, I will reply something like this,
'I'd tell them they are enough. I would tell them that everyone has knock backs and everyone has moments that didn't work out and that they should not allow the difficult days of the past steal a potential

future from them. I'd tell them their sense of inadequacy is lying to them.'

That's exactly what I would say because I've heard myself saying those words to people on numerous occasions. Yet, as I give that advice and listen to my own voice saying those words, I am keenly aware of my hypocrisy, but rather than take my own advice, I have chosen to add being a hypocrite to what I should be ashamed of.

When I first started a course of talking therapy, my counsellor suggested that I create a practice of self-affirmation. Within the first 45 minutes of my first session with her, she had helped me name the complex system of shame that had entangled my mind. As long as that complex was left unaddressed, we agreed, I would find progress and recovery in my mental health would be extremely slow work.

Marriage experts speak of the 'magic ratio' of interactions a couple had with one another. This concept combining from research[4] carried out by Drs. John Gottman and Robert Levenson concluded that, within healthy relationships, for every negative interaction a couple

---

4

https://www.gottman.com/blog/the-magic-relationship-ratio-according-science/

has they must have five positive interactions. This ratio helps the couple to hold a healthy view of one another and their relationship.

I often wonder if that same magic ratio works on the relationship we have with ourselves. Would our mental health and self-esteem improve drastically if for every self-critical or self-loathing thought that we have, we intentionally and consistently brought five positives thoughts about ourselves to mind? I don't know if the magic ratio of negative/positive interactions with ourselves would correlate exactly to the magic ratio within marriages but after following my counsellor's guidance and creating a practice of self-affirmation I am sure that choosing a 1:5 ratio has the potential to be transformational for anyone.

Cards on the table; self-affirmation was extremely uncomfortable for me at first. I was advised, against anything that felt natural to me, to speak positive affirmations about myself, out loud, as I looked in the mirror every morning. I was to ask myself certain questions and answer them with only positive answers. Here are some of those questions.

Who am I looking at?
What am I good at?

What do I see when I look at my own face?

Who will be happy to see me today?

What part of who I am and I proud of today?

On day one of this practice (a practice, by the way, which I felt was a waste of time but was so desperate for peace of mind that I was willing to give a try) I felt awkward and embarrassed as I told my reflection my own name, that I thought I was good at baking bread and that my mother would be glad to see me. I failed to answer any other questions. I think the other two affirmations I gave myself were that my shirt was good and something about not being the worst singer on earth. Honestly, that first day, my new habit of being positive about myself had no positive effect that I was aware of but I stuck with it. Every day for weeks, I would look in the mirror and tell myself good things about the person looking back at me.

The first time I noticed that it was having an effect was when I heard myself say that I was good at something when talking to other people. Anyone who knows me will tell you that one of my worst habits is self-deprecation. The majority of the time I do it because I find it funny, but I do it to a fault and anybody with a shred of social intelligence will realise that at times, it is not a joke, but is a betrayal of low self-esteem. Hearing myself publicly affirm my own ability was the first moment I realised that practising self-affirmation was working, I was beginning to untangle the shame that had been holding me back.

At a later session with my counsellor I was asked this question;
What do you think you could achieve if you were not held back by shame?

This question was the first time I had begun to imagine what a life outside of the confines of my own self-shaming could look like? Not only was it possible that I could become more positive about my day to day life as it was, but I could actually begin to imagine things that I could work towards that I would have previously disqualified myself from. At the time, I replied that I would apply for a promotion within the organisation I was working for at the time. Three months earlier I would have talked myself out of applying for any number reasons, all of which boiled down to shame. I applied, I got the job. Things began to move forward.

I soon found myself directly addressing the thoughts, words and events that had linked together to form that complex of shame in my mind. I began to name as lies, the times which other people had told me I was worth less than I am. I told myself the truth that the memories of shaming moments most likely only survived in my own mind and they did not deserve another second of my life. I began the process of dismantling the shame complex I had built, one moment at a time. I was able to begin redefining my shaming experiences and so lessened their power over me.

Don't be mistaken, this is no fairytale ending. I still find myself regularly falling back into self-loathing. I still allow people to speak to me and treat me in ways that I would never allow them to do to other people. I accept mistreatment and being undermined all too regularly. I still allow shame to silence my voice when I should speak. The difference is that now I realise I am doing it, and I respond by taking steps to change my behaviour or to retrospectively defend myself or to change the negative narrative about who I am that I have allowed to develop. I have many miles left to travel but I've come so far already.

What would your life look like if the words of shame that you think and speak about yourselves were replaced by positive affirmation? What choices would you have made differently had you not been held back by a sense of shame? Who would you stop from mistreating you if you could overcome the shame which tells you their actions are justified?

What are your answers to the five questions above? Who do you see in the mirror? What is that person good at? What do you see when you look at their face? What makes you proud of yourself? Who is delighted that you are alive? Do the experiment that I did. Ask yourself those questions every morning starting tomorrow. Positive answers only.

I believe that speaking positive truths to ourselves has a powerful effect. I believe that disciplining ourselves to be self-affirming, rapidly disempowers our sense of shame and the person who we always hoped we could be begin to emerge. I also believe that speaking positively to ourselves also enables us to speak positively to others. Positivity attracts positivity. Do not be surprised if your practice of self-affirmation results in affirmation from others. People will begin to notice your rising self-esteem. People will notice your willingness to step forward.

As ridiculous as I felt when I first started my practice, I cannot deny the difference it has made. I regularly find myself doing things which I could not have imagined myself doing before I started. I am more confident, less willing to accept mistreatment and much more willing to put myself forward for things I believe I am capable of. I hope, that if you too have been held back by shame, that you can begin to unravel it. I hope that you can one day soon find yourself free from shame, living a life filled with taken opportunities and celebration.

## 8. Expectations

I can remember my first day of school very clearly. I was one of those kids who happily skipped into the classroom without looking back. I can remember the bumpy red fabric of my school tie and the uncomfortable shirt around my scrawny, little neck.

Two things stand out from that day. The first is that I got to paint with a lot of red paint and a man from the paper came and took my photograph as I painted. My first day at school and I was already being hounded by the media. The other thing I remember is that the boy next to me bit the boy on the other side of him and was whisked off to the principal. I don't know what happened to him that day but I have found myself worried that he was subjected to some form of physical punishment. Corporal punishment in schools became illegal the following year. I hope he wasn't. Being physically harmed on your first day in school serves only to cause long term difficulty in one's relationship with education.

The first day done, and I was off; another soul dropped into the river of education. There was no getting out of the water now for at least 12 years. My peers and I would spend the rest of our childhoods being assessed and reassessed, tested and challenged. We would be graded and streamed based upon verbal reasoning and handwriting. We would split into groups of grammar school qualifiers and comprehensive school qualifiers. We would meet with careers advisors and we would meet with army recruiters. We would fill in a survey for something called JigCal and then find out we were a perfect match for a career in either operatic stage management or dry stone walling. We would pass exams and fail exams and move up a set or down a set.

We would wait for an envelope in August to tell us if we were to be welcomed back to the school for more of the same, and we would choose apprenticeships and skills training and go out to build businesses. We would have sleepless nights before exams and we would write personal statements about being driven self-starters. We would wait for offers and rejections from universities and we would nervously take our first customers to our trade. We would wait again two August's later for another letter to come. We would have that one last party with our friends before packing our lives into a car and moving into halls of residence and student houses for it all to start again at university. We'd study, we'd learn, we'd grow up, we'd graduate, we'd get jobs, we'd meet someone, we'd break up, we'd meet someone else and some of us would get married. Someone would get divorced and then another one.

We'd change jobs and emigrate to other countries and start our own companies and work for our family firms. We would buy flats and then houses with gardens. We'd start to have our first children and then our seconds and sometimes even more. We'd talk about which school was best for them and where the best parks were.

Then all of a sudden we would wake up and we'd be almost 40. We'd suddenly be much older than our teachers were on our first days of school. Our kids are the ones skipping off happily into the classroom or clinging to thighs crying to go home. Our kids are the ones biting one another and being whisked out of the room. Our kids are painting for the cameras. The cycle starts again. We have barely caught our breath. Life rushed on and we kept rushing with it.

I am happy with where I am now but I look at the system we have in place and it feels like our educational and career paths are set out for us even before we start primary school. We are like a coin dropped into the slot of one of those penny drop machines (nobody knows their real name) at a seaside amusements arcade. We fall through the slot and the machine takes us on the path it chooses. We are knocked one way and then the other until we land with the other coins that took the same course. There are no exit ramps and no pit stops, we study for 12, 14 or even 21 years and then we work for 40 years or more. We do make choices, but it often seems like we are caught in a current and we don't even consider trying to swim against it until one day it throws us out into the ocean of the big bad world.

That big bad world, of course, comes with its own sets of expectations and those sets will compete with one another for our time and our energy. We've developed language and strategies for helping us to cope with these competing draws upon our lives; systems to help us survive the tension. We call it work-life balance and in doing so compartmentalise our lives into two sides which will compete for our attention. For every must-attend meeting that runs past 6 pm is a must-attend meal with our families. For every work trip away is a series of missed bedtime stories and cuddles with our kids.

This is how it has been for over 100 years and since the dawn of the internet, it seems to have only gotten worse. The internet was designed to make our jobs easier, and for a long time, did, speeding up communication across the globe and building more efficient businesses and organisations. I imagine that the initial surge in email use made a lot of people's jobs less stressful and created space in their lives. Then we realised that faster communication creating space in our diaries meant that our workload capacity increased.

When I first got email I received a maximum of two emails a day. This morning I woke up to 54 new messages, the majority are marketing emails but the number of communications we send and receive is dangerously excessive. I am convinced that a slow fused mental health crisis began when our workforce cultures began to change to expect email to exponentially increase output.

The pressure to deliver ramped up. Work tasks could suddenly go home with anyone who had a home computer or laptop. Work that was once reliant on post office and a mail trolley could now be delivered from anywhere with an internet connection and at any time of the day. One by one we began to feel the expectations placed upon us grow heavier and heavier. Email meant more could be done, so we had to give more.

Then, in 2007 the iPhone arrived and expectations went even further into overdrive. Communication that was once limited to a building with an internet connection could now be in every worker's pocket. Even more, work could be produced. Work could now be done at any time, anywhere in the world. Email was now portable and always with us.

The last 13 years have seen us continually adding the management and administration of new apps and platforms to our personal and professional labour. We are dealing with communication across any number of systems at any one time. We throw millions of words a minute out into the world on social media. We scroll through photos of our friends' lives, clicking a heart for the people we like the most. We watch silly dances and lip-syncs. We sell things and we review things.

The pace of life, both at work and in the rest of our existence, has increased dramatically in the past two decades and it has been exhausting. If I could point to one thing that triggers panic and anxiety in me it is the frantic and frenetic pace of life. I am unable to cope with the incessant bombardment of information. I do not have the emotional resilience to process the horrors of the world that find their way from the palm of my hand into my brain in live HD. My brain is not able to cope with a news feed on an app that seamlessly moves from wedding photos to terrorism to a new baby to fake news to protests to cookery to jokes to a pandemic.

I just want to scream, 'STOP! SOMEONE, PLEASE MAKE IT STOP!' We don't need to go faster, we don't need to do more, we don't need new platforms. I cannot keep up. If I try it's going to make me very ill. I need an off-ramp. I cannot keep up with the expectation to function at this pace across so many plains. I need it to stop. I think a lot of us do. Yet, for some reason that I don't understand, I keep logging in. I keep checking emails. I keep trying new apps. Perhaps I am addicted. Perhaps we all are.

In his excellent book, The Growth Delusion[5], David Pilling lays out an argument that the western world has bought in wholesale to the idea that economic growth is what will lead to health and well-being. He shows, that in the initial faces of these kinds of society, as GDP rises so does well-being, people eat healthier, sanitation systems improve, access to healthcare increases and so, therefore, does well-being. Yet, it is not an eternal correlation, for at some point the relationship between economic growth and well-being breaks down. The economy continues to grow but the well-being line plateaus and then goes into reverse. His argument, an economy growing at the expense of the health of the citizens it serves is damaging to our lives. It is an excellent book and well worth reading.

Yesterday, we spent the day with a group of friends helping my dear friend Mark do some gardening on the land of the retreat centre he manages. We cut hedges, dug flower beds and pulled out tree stumps as the kids played on the grass nearby. The only sounds we could hear were the sounds of hedge clippers, branches falling, the scrape of a spade and children laughing. At one stage I walked to another part of the land to get a different tool and the lack of electronic and human

---

5

https://www.bloomsbury.com/uk/the-growth-delusion-9781408893722/

noise was beautiful. Nature was far from silent, but the noise it made was soothing. It was in complete contrast to how my normal life can feel sometimes. I was not rushed, I was not bombarded, I was calm and at peace.

My mind is haunted by the voice of expectation. I look back and feel that for years I was out of control of where I was going and just went with the current of the educational system. For years further I, driven by how I felt I was meant to behave, allowed myself to be torn apart by competing expectations. It is only now at the age of 39 that I'm unwilling to do that anymore.

I need to make changes. I need to say no more often. I need to work hard for the hours I am employed and come home to my family. I need to spend more time doing very little with the people I love. I need to be willing to risk letting people down for the sake of my own health. I need to let the latest controversial topic on social media pass me by without drawing my engagement. I need to stop reading the comments section. I need to unfollow and block voices that cause me anxiety. I need to leave the house without my phone and go to the woods or get in the sea.

I need to change because I can't do it anymore. I need to change because I don't want to miss my sons' childhoods because I am too busy looking at my phone. I need to change because my wife's face is much more wonderful than anything Instagram can show me.

The voice of expectation that pushes me to do these things is born in the fear of missing out and the fear of being less than I can be. The best I can be is to be there for those who need me most and in turn, they are the best thing for me. I need to choose them.

If you can see yourself here, then join me in changing. I don't think we will hit the end of our lives and be delighted about being exhausted from chasing after real or imagined expectations. We will regret not seeing the faces of our loved ones more often. Make a choice now before something else comes along and ramps the pace up again. We get to say no. It's an excellent little word. Use it more.

## 9. Why?

At some point, in the thousands of years of human history, people began to understand their lives as stories and themselves as the main protagonists of those stories. It is, of course, only natural that once our species developed the ability to tell stories which bound our ancestors together into tribes with shared history and cultures, that it would follow that we would begin to understand our lives in the same way.

As oral traditions passed down their tales of gods and ancestors through cultures, the stories we told one another became littered with narratives in which things work together in the end, sometimes for the person in the story, and sometimes for their descendants. The mythology of ancient cultures consistently tells of events, even when filled with terror and destruction, combining for the good of the protagonists and their people.

In the sacred documents of the major world religions, the stories take another step forward, suffering becomes purposed, pain becomes purposed, every dark event is a step towards something good. God works in mysterious ways and when we face trials we should open our eyes to understand that the trial is for our benefit.

Many of the great authors of the past 300 years filled their books with the same idea that no event in the protagonist's life is a mistake or to be wasted, but are instead all leading them towards the triumphant crescendo. The blockbuster movies and television shows of the 20th and 21st centuries take joy in delivering a twist in the last third of the film, turning deep tragedy to triumph for the star who saves the day, gets the girl, or wins the war.

After thousands of years of stories in which every event reported is there for the higher purpose as dreamed up by the storyteller, it is natural that we should begin to view our lives through the same lens. Thousands of years of turning the lives of our ancestors and mythical heroes into these kinds of narratives will naturally lead to us unconsciously believing that the stories in which we are the protagonists are written towards the same happily-ever-after endings.

This plays out in ways that we will all feel familiar with. It is seen when faced with a difficult choice between two options, we throw our energies and effort into the choice we make and if it turns out to be successful, assure ourselves that we made the right choice and it was meant to be. Would we have had less success had we made a different choice? Would our hard work have paid off less on the other option? We don't know that we wouldn't be seeing better results from the other choice and therefore declaring that it, in fact, was meant to be.

We also, conversely, find ourselves making choices the results of which are painful or disappointing and telling ourselves the other choice would have been better. We tell ourselves we missed the right choice. Again, we have no idea if that is true, but our minds, disciplined from our culture of storytelling, believe that in every choice there is a good and bad path, so if we are experiencing a bad result, we must have chosen the bad path.

Of course life does not work that way. Sometimes things go wrong that have nothing to do with whether you made the right choice or not. Sometimes any choice would be a good choice and other times any choice would lead to a painful result. Life is not a video game through which there is one pathway. It is a series of millions of decisions and happenstance that lead us to both good and bad places and it is almost impossible to create a coherent, purposed storyline from those decisions.

The urge to ask 'why?' and the need to know why things happen in my life has caused me heartache that I could have avoided. The need to find some sort of higher or divine purpose in the most painful events in my life increased my pain as I played things over and over in my mind, in the vain hope of seeing some detail that revealed an unfolding plan. The pains of broken relationships, rejection, bereavement and illness cause their own pain, my insistence on trying to find out why those things happened was like inviting that pain to set up permanent residence in the forefront of my mind.

Searching for a reason why every painful thing that has happened to me did happen, has driven to long periods of depression and anxiety. Sifting through these things has done anything but bring any sense of peace, it has stirred up turmoil as there is more often than not, no answer to the question I am asking. The best answer to the question 'why?' that I have ever managed to muster up is that, 'life is hard and bad things happen.' What a disappointing answer.

As I've begun to try and curb my need for a purpose to my pain I've realised just how harmful the idea that suffering has to have a purpose can be. It steals from us the ability to engage properly with grief. It slows down or even halts our movement towards healing from our deepest wounds. The search for a reason causes us to linger at the scene of our pain, frozen where we were wounded, waiting for something to change. We don't move on quickly. We don't rebuild as quickly. We tarry in anticipation of an answer that is never going to come. The false hope will break our hearts a second time.

The question 'why?' lives next door to the even less kind question, 'Why me?' 'Why me?' rarely leads to an answer that doesn't devalue our worth. I have thrown myself headlong into that question and without exception ended up creating a story that tells me that I deserve to be hurt.

I am yet to meet anyone (they may exist) who asks 'why me?' in the face of great suffering and comes up with an answer that doesn't heap blame on top of pain. When we crave an answer to why me, we tend towards redefining the worst results of the chaos of life on earth as punishment for our failures, shortcomings or sins. That path will only lead us to misery. We are already in pain, we are already in grief, we do not need to amplify those things with self-loathing.

The most useful practice I have discovered when trying to stop asking why is to begin to phrase these moments in my life as factual statements and creative or productive questions. 'Why did he have to die?' has no answer, it has no outcome. Questions like, 'He died, how do I remember life without him?' or 'he died, how can I honour him in my life?' lead to outcomes and thoughts about the future. They cause us to move beyond the stagnating waters of where we are towards somewhere new.

Changing 'why?' to 'what now?' has helped me to stop dwelling in the dark moments and to begin to move towards, not just healing, but to living well beyond the pain. I realise this sounds like semantics or wordplay, but the reality is that we experience nothing of the world except in our minds and we must learn to discipline our minds towards ways of thinking that give us life rather than take life from us.

Not every event has a lesson. Some wounds we will never heal from but we learn to live with them and we will never be the same again. Some grief will live long in our souls. We will never know why. There is, however, always an answer to 'what now?' The immediate answer might be to cry your heart out until you're ready to think about a future. The answer might be to get a therapist or to go on medication. The answer might be to dust yourself off and keep on trying. There will be always an answer to what now.

'What now?' created hope that even if my walk through life was slowed by a burden of grief at least I was still moving. 'What now?' let me believe that out of the wreckage of divorce that new love and even a family might exist. 'What now?' told me that a career lost might lead me into a new career in which I would feel even more fulfilled.

Be kind to yourself, stop hurting yourself by asking 'why?' You deserve better than that. You deserve a future. You deserve a life beyond grief, pain and blame. You deserve to feel joy again. These things have happened, that won't change. What is next for you?

# A Moment of Pause 2: Counselling

'No, I'm okay I think, I don't think I need counselling. Thanks for caring enough to suggest it though. I appreciate it.' There will be more than one person reading this who might remember me saying that to them. Others will remember me saying, 'I've actually had a lot of time to process this stuff on my own and it has been good for me.'

I knew for a long time that I needed some help. I had got so caught up in my own negative thoughts that I was regularly spiralling in private. I was sure I was holding it all together in public. I was not and more and more people started to suggest I talk to someone. I eventually had a significant panic attack in a meeting and decided that enough was enough. I needed to overcome my own nervousness, embarrassment and fear, and get some help

I could not put a finger on one thing that caused the decline in my mental health and that made me nervous about calling to arrange an appointment. The reality was, my illness was down to the fact that I'd failed to process a lot of things for a long time. I had plodded on with a mix of stubbornness, denial and a stiff upper lip. Nothing ruins your mental health quite like trying to be stoic does.

The morning after that panic attack I dropped my son off at his nursery school and pulled into a car park to call the number of a counselling agency. I held my phone in my hand for 25 minutes before I called the number. I can remember sweating with nerves. It took a monumental effort to make that call. When I did eventually call, I can recall the weakness in my shaky voice as I explained why I was calling.

I am telling you this because I think that is a lot of people's experience of seeking help with their mental health. There is a tightrope to walk between knowing you are ill and need assistance, and the fact that admitting that will make it all seem even more real, and that in itself is terrifying. In my experience of that reluctance to make the call, there was also a real sense that I might get it wrong, or I might not actually be as ill as I felt. I feared that I would lose control of the conversation and end up being forced to address things before I was ready. I found a hundred reasons to talk myself out of calling until the reason that meant I needed to make the call was getting out of hand.

Ten days later I pulled up in a different car park and walked into a waiting room. My name was called and I sat down opposite a small woman of about 50. My first thought was that she looked kind. She had a quiet voice and I was really aware that she moved very deliberately and gently. The room was plain and the seat was one of those leather tub chairs from Ikea. Her chair was different. I asked her if that was deliberate. It wasn't, she hired the room.

I remember as I sat down I couldn't stop  thinking about Tony Soprano. I laughed to myself about the way that my mind works and then the first session started. It was nothing like I expected it to be at all.

The first five minutes were basic introductions, who I was, what I did for a living, etc. It was the type of thing you talk to someone about when you're sitting next to them on a flight and they haven't taken your earbuds being in as a hint. It was a very relaxed conversation.

Then, without missing a beat the counsellor asked me why I thought I should get counselling. Her voice didn't change, her demeanour remained the same. She somehow managed to make the question as unintimidating as the previous questions had been.

'I'm falling apart and I need help. I don't love myself. I think I have little to offer and the things I do have to offer, I believe that nobody would ever want.'

I winced a little at my honesty. I didn't expect to open up that quickly, so I told her that.

'Wow. I didn't think I'd be that open. You're good at this,' I said.
'I guess you are more ready than you thought you were,' was her reply.

Over the sessions I had in that room I talked about things I'd never talked about. I remembered the details of events that I had long forgotten but could still remember the pain of. It was good to talk. It was good to get things out of my mind that had been rattling around in there for a long time. It was liberating to acknowledge my complete lack of self-worth out loud. It felt for the first time that naming that would have no negative consequence.

At some point during the second session, I realised that I wasn't actually having a conversation with the counsellor. I was talking to myself. She was there just to guide me as I spoke to myself about who I was, what I was afraid of and how much I was hurting. I spoke and I listened. I gave words to feelings that had never been spoken of before and as I did I came to know myself better.

I would begin to talk about something and the counsellor would wait for a natural pause and then draw me back to a phrase or sentence that I had said. She would ask me to explain what I meant, or would ask a question that caused me to think about that phrase from another angle. These questions allowed me to uncover things that I'd hidden under defence mechanisms and denial.

She didn't once ask about my father.

I would be sent home with work to do. I have already mentioned the creation of a practice of self-affirmation. It felt so hard at first but it worked. I would be asked to consider how I could say no to things I didn't want to and was supposed to say no to at least three things per week. I failed for two weeks in a row. I was asked to be honest with certain people about how I felt about things.

Everything I was asked to do, with the exception of the affirmation practice, felt very natural and normal to me. A lot of it was common sense advice that I had given to other people. The hard part was putting it into practice or believing that I was a person who needed to hear that advice.

At the end of each session, I would say thanks, shake her hand and go and buy a coffee to drink on the drive home. On two occasions I spilled it over my jeans.

Nothing I was asked to do was weird. I didn't at any stage feel set upon or under pressure. I didn't feel trapped or cornered. My greatest fears about counselling were all shown to be unnecessary fears. It was nothing like what you see on tv. It felt really normal and comfortable.

The common wisdom is that it can sometimes take a while to find a counsellor who feels like a good match for you. It is important that there is some kind of chemistry between you and your counsellor that enables that natural and free-flowing conversation to occur. I was very fortunate that the first person I spoke to I felt was really suitable. That may not happen though, you should try a few if the first one doesn't feel like the right fit. This is common practice and counsellors will be used to it. You don't have to worry about offending them. It would be frustrating for them if you went with them and it didn't work because you were not the right fit.

If you're aware that you need counselling and have fears about what it would be like, I can reassure you that it is not something to be fearful of. I am also very happy to answer any questions about this via twitter

@davemagill. My DMs are always open. If talking to me about counselling puts your mind at ease just enough to go and talk to someone then I am more than happy to talk.

## 10.   A life worth living

As a child, I loved the film, The Wizard of Oz, even though I distinctly remember being scared of the Wicked Witch ('I'm melting'). There is a moment in that film when Dorothy and Toto are caught up into the whirlwind and carried out of Kansas to another world. That moment, where she leaves the storm and enters this other place coincides with the cinematography changing from black and white to glorious 1930s technicolour. I am sure when that movie was first released this was a powerful moment for those watching. By the time I was first watching the film in the 1980s, colour television was the norm, there was no gasp at its appearance. I wish I could have experienced that film in that authentic way and felt the excitement of that change.

I think that moment of the film is a good illustration of what my experience with coming out of the darkness of the most difficult periods with my mental health has been like. The contrast between the violence of a storm, the fear, the darkness and the lack of colour with the happiness, songs and fantastic creatures of Oz is not dissimilar to the contrast between my mental health declining and my recovery.

Anxiety and depression took the colour out of my world. It made me lethargic. I lacked any desire to achieve or try anything. It made me uninterested in my relationships, trapped by the idea that I would be rejected in the end, so trying now was pointless. I couldn't but was constantly drowsy and exhausted. I lost my appetite but put on weight from over-eating bad food. I couldn't enjoy anything properly but instead found fault or drifted into my own mind and missed what happened around me.

When I think of what I was like at my lowest ebb I think about asking The Pope or Archbishop of Canterbury to consider canonising my wife. She carried me through months of our relationship with very little ever coming back to her. Anxiety and depression created in me a self-obsession that would have felt like selfishness to anyone around me. I am sure I was a drain down which her love and care were often washed without me ever showing her the appreciation she deserved.

Whilst all of this was happening I lived in denial that there was anything wrong. I refused to accept that any of the voices in my head, as discussed in this book, existed. I was fine. I could cope. I was strong enough. I needed help but refused to see that I did. I refused to get help, that is, until I had no choice. My body began to give up the fight and that collapse forced me to stop pretending.

That life was not the life that I wanted to live. It was dull and painful. I was not suicidal and I am thankful I didn't have to deal with that, but I was miserable. Life could be so much more. I needed to feel and taste and see colour again. I needed to sleep better. I missed the connection with other people. I was physically present but emotionally absent. I was lost in my own life. I needed escape or rescue. I was desperate.

I wish I could say that life turned to colour with the same speed as a Hollywood scene change can. It didn't, but every day, the hue of my world changed a little bit. Things changed for the brighter. Things got better. I began to hope again as I crawled my way back from the edge.

The things I've talked about in the chapters of this book were not easy wins, nor are they some kind of magical formula. I cannot promise that if you choose to try the same things that they will work, but I definitely believe you should try them. In particular, if you recognise that you are unwell, you should reach out to someone who can help.

That might be a friend, a colleague, a GP or a therapist. Please reach out to someone.

The thing I can say that I am sure helps everyone, is building a disciplined approach to good mental wellbeing. Practices of, for example, self-affirmation and changing 'why? to 'what next?' will not cure mental illness but they will help you dilute the intensity of your pain. Some of us may not, no matter how hard we try, be able to overcome our brain chemistry and will need the help of medication. That is the situation I am in at the moment. I need that little pill to help me through the day, but that pill is supported in its work by better self-care,the discipline of my thoughts towards positivity and speaking truth in the face of lies. These things combined have made a world of difference.

I have noticed that a lot of the people I know who walk a similar trail to me in this area came to seek help too late. Almost all of them delayed seeking help because they deemed themselves not worth helping. For some this meant that they viewed themselves of such low value that they didn't deserve help. For others, it meant that they thought their pain was not significant enough. For others, they felt that they were too strong to need help. This is a trap of mental illness. Our ability to disqualify ourselves from help is what can keep us suffering. It holds us fast in a dark place and stops us from seeking rescue.

You are worth it. You have talent and wonder within you. You have words that need to be heard and love that needs to be shared. You have people whose world you light up when they see you, and people who are delighted you exist. You will create and you will celebrate. You will laugh and laugh some more. There is joy still to be found. You are worth helping. You're not being selfish in seeking it. You're not a drama king or queen. You're not deserving of pain. You're worth it. You're precious. You're wonderful.

If you are suffering at the hands of your own mind, and have felt some resonance with this book, then please ask for help. You won't regret it. I promise. Don't let your own mind keep itself trapped in pain. There are ways out of this. They may not be easy, but they are out there.

# Appendix 1: Affirmations for every week of the year.

As I mentioned earlier in this book, one of the things I found hardest in building a practice of self-care was affirming myself. It was just the awkwardness of looking at myself in the mirror and speaking positively. It was that I didn't know where to begin. I found it really hard to come up with anything to say.

Below are 52 affirmations which you can speak to your own mind. If you can find the strength to believe these statements about yourself, you will begin to experience a difference in your through patterns. You may begin to experience better self-esteem and a more positive outlook.

Some of these statements will deconstruct your sense of failure and some will build up your willingness to accept help. Some of these statements will encourage you to push yourself towards opportunity and some will affirm you in the place where you are now.

I suggest you work through one a week, focussing on that affirmation every day for 7 days, then repeat this for the next one, but remember to continue to regularly affirm yourself in the previous statements. This does not need to a long drawn out affair, five minutes or so before you get in the shower, or before you get out of the car at the office. As the weeks progress, think around the statements you are making, state the evidence from your life that proves the statement to be true. I've left some spaces for you to write one piece of evidence per day.

In choosing to affirm yourself and to consider the evidence that shows the affirmation to be true, you will begin to change the tone in which you view yourself. You may even begin to like yourself. Choosing to love ourselves and to acknowledge the good things about ourselves is a life-giving experience.

**52 Statements of Affirmation.**

1. My pain is real.

   a.

   b.

   c.

   d.

   e.

   f.

   g.

2. My voice is worth listening to.

   a.

   b.

   c.

   d.

   e.

   f.

   g.

3. My work is worthwhile.

    a.

    b.

    c.

    d.

    e.

    f.

    g.

4. I am loved and loveable.

    a.

    b.

    c.

    d.

    e.

    f.

    g.

5. My body can do amazing things.

    a.

    b.

    c.

    d.

    e.

    f.

g.

6. My opinions are valid.

   a.

   b.

   c.

   d.

   e.

   f.

   g.

7. Even at my , I am still worthy.

   a.

   b.

   c.

   d.

   e.

   f.

   g.

8. I don't have to accept other people's mistreatment of me.

   a.

   b.

   c.

   d.

   e.

f.

g.

9. My ability to produce has no bearing upon my value.

   a.

   b.

   c.

   d.

   e.

   f.

   g.

10. My life is worth celebrating.

    a.

    b.

    c.

    d.

    e.

    f.

    g.

11. My failures do not define me.

    a,

    b.

    c.

    d.

e.

f.

g.

12. I can do more than I imagine.

a.

b.

c.

d.

e.

f.

g.

13. My dreams are worth pursuing.

a.

b.

c.

d.

e.

f.

g.

14. I am beautiful.

a.

b.

c.

d.

e.

f.

g.

15. I have made mistakes less often than I've got things right.

a.

b.

c.

d.

e.

f.

g.

16. When I show kindness it makes a difference.

a.

b.

c.

d.

e.

f.

g.

17. I am significant to more people than I think I am.

a.

b.

c.

d.

e.

f.

g.

18. People want to know who I really am.

a.

b.

c.

d.

e.

f.

g.

19. Other people's expectations do not define me.

a.

b.

c.

d.

e.

f.

g.

20. My feeling of loneliness is valid.

a.

b.

c.

d.

e.

f.

g.

21. Self-care is not selfish.

a.

b.

c.

d.

e.

f.

g.

22. It is healthy to choose rest.

a.

b.

c.

d.

e.

f.

g.

23. Saying no sometimes is good for me.

    a.

    b.

    c.

    d.

    e.

    f.

    g.

24. I have good things in my life to celebrate.

    a.

    b.

    c.

    d.

    e.

    f.

    g.

25. My health is more important than my weight.

    a.

    b.

    c.

    d.

    e.

    f.

g.

26. I can give my trust at my own pace.

     a.

     b.

     c.

     d.

     e.

     f.

     g.

27. My security is worth protecting.

     a.

     b.

     c.

     d.

     e.

     f.

     g.

28. I have many good days ahead of me.

     a.

     b.

     c.

     d.

     e.

f.

g.

29. I am no more or less than anybody else.

   a.

   b.

   c.

   d.

   e.

   f.

   g.

30. Many small positive changes can change my life.

   a.

   b.

   c.

   d.

   e.

   f.

   g.

31. My generosity makes a difference to the lives of others.

   a.

   b.

   c.

   d.

e.

f.

g.

32. I do not need to understand why I have been hurt.

a.

b.

c.

d.

e.

f.

g.

33. My worst days are rarely connected to one another.

a.

b.

c.

d.

e.

f.

g.

34. I get to choose who takes up my time.

a.

b.

c.

d.

e.

f.

g.

35. I can walk away from toxic relationships.

a.

b.

c.

d.

e.

f.

g.

36. I did not deserve to be treated badly.

a.

b.

c.

d.

e.

f.

g.

37. Taking mediation doesn't lessen my value.

a.

b.

c.

d.

e.

f.

g.

38. The cruel words of others no power over my future.

a.

b.

c.

d.

e.

f.

g.

39. I am stronger than I think I am.

a.

b.

c.

d.

e.

f.

g.

40. I am able to succeed.

    a.

    b.

    c.

    d.

    e.

    f.

    g.

41. Comparing myself to other people will ruin my day.

    a.

    b.

    c.

    d.

    e.

    f.

    g.

42. I deserve help when I need it.

    a.

    b.

    c.

    d.

    e.

    f.

g.

43. It is my right to remove myself from damaging situations.

a.

b.

c.

d.

e.

f.

g.

44. My healing is more important than the expectations of others.

a.

b.

c.

d.

e.

f.

g.

45. Time spent on my own joy and pleasure is vital. It is not selfish.

a.

b.

c.

d.

e.

f.

g.

46. I will not give more time to those who have already abused the time I've given them.

a.

b.

c.

d.

e.

f.

g.

47. I can always decide what happens next?

a.

b.

c.

d.

e.

f.

g.

48. I have insight that is worth sharing.

a.

b.

c.

d.

e.

f.

g.

49. I am not disqualified by my life story.

a.

b.

c.

d.

e.

f.

g.

50. Spending time and money on my own joy is not greed.

a.

b.

c.

d.

e.

f.

g.

51. Doing what I love is not wasting my life even if it not what others would do.

    a.

    b.

    c.

    d.

    e.

    f.

    g.

52. I will not give up on my recovery.

    a.

    b.

    c.

    d.

    e.

    f.

    g.

## Appendix 2: How to get help from your GP.

I am sure that a lot of people never make the call to their GP because they are nervous and do not know what to say. This leads to them suffering longer than they need to. Here is some advice on how to get help from your doctor

:

- The phone call to arrange the appointment feels huge to you, to the receptionist taking the call it is a run of the mill diary booking. This will result in a mismatch of feeling on the call. Expect that and don't let it confuse you when it happens.
- Your GP speaks to a lot of patients about their mental health. They will not be shocked by you, they will not judge you. This is something they are very used to. Again, this will feel at odds with how you feel about the appointment. Try and bring yourself to their energy level as best you can. Draw from their calm.
- Write down what you plan to say. In the moment it will feel easy to avoid saying how you feel. The emotions of seeking help can sometimes cause us to downplay our symptoms. Having them written down in advance helps us to hold ourselves accountable to being honest about our situation.

- Write down your symptoms and their severity. Write down how long you have been feeling this way. Write down anything that you think exacerbates or triggers your illness.
- Be prepared to be asked if you have considered hurting yourself. This is normal. It can feel accusatory but it is part of the normal procedure for a doctor. Be honest in your answer.
- Write down what you hope the outcomes of the appointment will be. If you want to start medication or receive guidance on where to receive therapy then have notes to remind you to share those desires with the doctor.
- If you think it would make a difference to whether or not you will seek help, it is acceptable to have someone accompany you to the appointment. If you do have someone join you I advise that they take simple notes of what is said and what the doctor suggests. It is very easy for an anxious mind to miss those details because they are caught up in the stress of the moment.
- It is likely that the GP will give you information about medical, therapeutic and non-treatment based help such as exercise plans or dietary advice. For example, it may be suggested that you consider cutting out stimulants such as caffeine from your diet. If there is a lot of information, ask for time to write it down before leaving the clinic.

- If you are given medication be sure to arrange and stick to any review schedule. It is possible that the first medication you are prescribed does not work perfectly for you or has too many side effects. It is important that you continue to discuss your medication with your GP to make sure the dosage and medication are correct. Again, keep a written record of the things you would wish to raise with the GP.
- If you think it would be helpful you can request copies of the GPs notes and a record of any advice about specific treatment options given by the doctor. Sometimes this gives a little peace of mind to those suffering from anxiety.
- It can be helpful to track and record your mood once you begin treatment. This will be helpful when you are reviewing your medication.

The key to keeping your anxiety about your first appointment low is preparation. When you are suffering in your mental health this preparation can be exhausting but that preparation will make the experience a lot more specific to your needs. Don't accept the thought that you are being a drain upon the doctor or that your questions are stupid. Being heard and having your questions answered will help you commit to your recovery.

## A small request from me.

I've published this book myself. I don't have a marketing budget or publishing house behind me. If you have found it helpful can I ask that you rate it on the site you bought it form or even consider writing a short review? This helps me get it out there.

If you are willing to share about it on your social media, (I'm pretty easy to find) please tag me in those posts and I will share your thoughts. I'll be hashtagging it on twitter with #TheThoughtsThatHauntUs. Again, this helps me get it out there.

Thank you for reading this and thank you for your support.

All the best
Dave

Printed in Great Britain
by Amazon